Battle for Sanity

My Journey With Fibromyalgia

Kara M. Ferris

Llumina Press

ISBN: 1-59526-617-8

Printed in the United States of America by Llumina Press

Library of Congress Control Number: 2006907796

Battle for Sanity

Dedication

With love, for Aloise.

To the memory of my beloved Grandpa Keith who struggled with me and gave me courage I wouldn't have found without him.

Introduction

A few weeks shy of my eighteenth birthday, I thought seventeen years, eleven months, and two weeks were all I could handle. I was at rock bottom, I couldn't breathe: I was suffocating and unable to think clearly.

The sun was shining, but I couldn't tell or even care. I knew tomorrow wasn't going to be a better day; I'd still be greeted with the same questions, same pain, same hollow explanations, the same frustration that was crushing me.

Cedar Bend Gold Course, green eight: I remember everything. Maybe I forced myself to remember how beautiful it was because I was thinking I might not ever be standing here, doing this, feeling this, again. The sunset was gorgeous, but I didn't, in the least bit, feel thankful to see it. I looked at my three companions, my brother and two close friends, and mused to myself at how innocent and unburdened they acted. Life appeared to be so easy for them. They had no idea the crazed and manic thoughts running through my head that very minute. They had no idea what I wanted to do, how desperately lonely I was even in their company.

Usually with these people I was calm and content. We always had a blast, but today was different. My mind was screaming inside my calm, confident posture. I couldn't stand there anymore. *I hate this*, I thought. *How can I be this unhappy?* I heard myself telling them my head hurt and I'd catch up with them later back at my house. I knew I was walking, but

I couldn't feel it. I felt dazed and slow. I started crying as soon as I knew they couldn't see me. *Am I crying?* Tears were falling down my face, but I didn't feel them. I didn't feel anything. I was thankful for and scared by my numbness. I got into my truck and drove, with no destination. I kept driving and didn't notice that I hadn't even turned on the radio.

I drove to a dead-end road overlooking an airport runway just outside of town. I watched the sunset; the bottom arch of the sun was just caressing the landscape. I couldn't suppress the lump that had settled in my throat. I didn't want to anymore. I cried in hiccup-y sobs that wracked my tiny frame. I was screaming and pounding on the steering wheel. I was a weak fraction of the person I'd once been, and it made me mad. I crawled down to the floor and curled up in a ball. I felt so pathetic but didn't care enough to try to change it. I wanted to die and prayed that God would just let me fall asleep and it would all be over. *Why isn't God here?* I hated Him and knew He didn't care what happened to me. *If you are real, give me a sign that you can hear me; show me that I'm not alone!* Nothing happened. I sat for what seemed like forever, and nothing happened. I was alone. I felt like nothing.

Chapter One

I *'m going to Grandma's.* That's all I could think. The words jumped into my head, casting away every other thought or hesitation. I don't know how long I'd been sitting at the end of that road, but it was late. The sun had set, and I hadn't even noticed. I picked myself up from the floor of the truck and drove home, determined. My brother was still golfing with our friends, and the rest of my family was at my other sister's softball game, so I returned home to just my little sister, the baby. I walked into the house, and she asked, "Kara what's wrong, why have you been crying?" I told her that I was going to go to Grandma's and that I was going to be fine. She just stared at me. I can't imagine what thoughts raced through her little head.

I went into my room, packed a small bag of the most random, weird things, and pulled my journal out of my dresser. I wasn't thinking clearly. I took two books, clothes for running but no running shoes, flip flops, and a huge sweater, although it was the middle of summer.

My sister came into my room and stood by the doorway. I told her that I was very sad and needed to see Grandma. I don't think she knew what to say. I wrote the weirdest note to my parents, telling them I was okay, that I wasn't running away from home, I wasn't suicidal, and that I just needed to get away. *I'm going to Grandmas*, I wrote. *I'll be fine. I love you. Don't let the kids worry.* I put the letter in the kitchen and gave the baby a hug. It broke my heart to leave her there alone. She looked at me like she was scared of me. I left my nine-year-old sister alone in our house—at night. Her big sister, the one she looked up to most in the world, just walked out and left her. I wonder what she did after I left. Cried? Called my parents? Nothing? What would any little girl do if her oldest sister said she was so sad she couldn't take it anymore and just left?

While I filled my gas tank, I took my first glance at the map. I had never made this long of a trip by myself—a four-hour drive and I was leaving at 9:30 in the evening. I didn't care. All that mattered was that I was leaving.

I cried, yelled, and prayed throughout the four hours it took to get there. I remember gripping the steering wheel in my clenched hands. I drove that way the whole time. I'd never driven with my hands like that before, and I haven't since. I stopped once halfway there to call my grandma. I didn't know if she was even in town. No one answered her phone, so I left a message and hoped for the best. My aunt lived two houses down, and two uncles lived in the same town. But I didn't have their phone numbers. I didn't even have a cell phone. I figured I could find somewhere to go. I was not, at all, in a clear state of mind. My guardian angel must have brought an entourage that night. I can't tell north from south if I'm looking at a compass, but I never got lost once and never got tired, even though I pulled in well after one the next morning.

My grandma was waiting up for me, with just the kitchen light on. I didn't say anything. I just collapsed on the couch, and my head fell into her lap. All I wanted to feel and think about were her tiny, pretty hands combing through my hair. She kept saying, "Honey, what happened? What's wrong? Please tell me what's wrong. We love you. Don't you know that?" For twenty minutes, I said nothing; I just cried. Finally, I looked up at her face and, for the second time that night, hated myself being the reason someone I loved looked so sad. I told her I'd just left, run away. I cried a waterfall until I had no more energy. She told me she had called my parents when she saw me pull up. "It's okay, honey. Let me put you to bed."

I slept well that night because I was so emotionally and physically exhausted. I woke up to someone saying, "Get up, beautiful." I opened my eyes to see my dad sitting in the chair next to my head. I asked him what he was doing there. He said he'd left right after he'd heard I'd split and had gotten there around 2:30 in the morning. Before he finished speaking, I was crying.

"Dad, I'm so sad. I feel like I'm dying inside, I need help, please." I begged him to fix me or find someone who would. I told him I couldn't go on this way and that the pain was making me crazy. "Dad, I'm so scared I'm going crazy. I can't think of anything else but the pain. There is no one to talk to. Nobody understands." I knew people wanted to, but nobody could. He promised he would do everything he could to make it better. I didn't believe it. I felt like he was another person just trying to get me to hold on for another day.

Chapter Two

I imagine this is what it feels like to live in a full suit of armor. My mind is fine, but no matter what I tell my body to do, it can't or won't do it. I just want to run, but I feel so heavy and slow. And I know that if I do, the next day I'll have to stay in bed all day. Just walking or getting out of a chair is hard sometimes. My body is so stiff, and I feel like my feet weigh a ton. My neck and shoulders always ache; my low back feels like knives are constantly poking it.

I'm not really living in a full suit of armor; I'm trapped in one. It's dark, and no matter what I do, I'm always cold. Maybe only I can hear it, but my body creeks every time I move. I'm too young to be living in this body. There must have been a mistake somewhere along the line. This isn't right. I have so many things I want to do, but my body can't keep up with my mind. I'm trapped. I'm a twenty-year-old living in an eighty-year-old woman's body!

For a long time, I felt like no one understood me. I guess I still feel like not many people understand me. Most of the time, I don't talk about how I feel physically because even though they try, nobody can understand. If someone tries to make light of my illness, I feel like I have to join in, despite my feelings. I try not to ask for help because I'm scared that when I really need it, my family and friends will be sick of hearing about my physical problems and won't want to help me anymore. I feel like no one in the world could be going through what I'm going through. Even worse, I've believed I was going crazy, and the very thought has paralyzed me with fear. Thinking about my pain and dealing with it makes me crazy, but I can't tell anyone. What if I *am* crazy?

There are a few reasons I wanted to write about my experiences. It's partly because it helps me to feel like I'm gaining control over this illness and mostly because I want other people with fibromyalgia to read this and know that they aren't alone, that they don't have to be scared. I want this to be something others with fibromyalgia can share with friends and family. I want to help others understand what we; as a fibromyalgia community are going through. Sometimes it's not easy to find the right words. Nothing that goes through our minds is abnormal. I promise, other people have thought it too. I know what it's like to feel weak and helpless. If nothing else, I want this book to be a comfort. Because for me, more than anything I just wanted someone to tell me that they believed me and that it wasn't all in my head. I didn't want to have to deal with the awful things doctors said to me by myself or have to feel like a loser or a failure because I was sick

Everyone has always tried to cheer me up and take my mind off my illness. But I can't take my mind off it; I have to think about it all the time. I always have to plan my day around how I'm feeling and consider the effects of my activities for the next day. Will this give me a headache? Can I afford to spend four extra hours in bed today?

I know what the looks are like from family and friends. I know how doctors treat us and I know the heartless things they can say. I know what it's like to have relationships ruined because of this. I've had my heart broken because some one I loved couldn't understand my illness or didn't want to try. I've wished I could be the normal girl they wanted. It has broken my heart to see the "will you just get better?" look on the faces of people I love. I've prayed that I wouldn't have to take so much medicine. I've worried about finding a man who can deal with me forever when I don't even know if I can deal with me forever.

I've included some thoughts from my loved ones about my illness. Those with fibromyalgia will recognize their loved ones in the voices of my family, I'm sure. I hope this is a book that they can share with people close to them. Maybe it will help explain things they can't quite explain themselves. Having support is so important, but they can't help you unless you let them. I'm thankful to have people that care about me and want to help me through this.

I believe that everything happens for a reason. I know that God gave me this challenge because he knew I could handle it. I don't always feel like I can, but some days I do. That's enough to keep me going. Fibromyalgia is going to be manageable one day. I'm sure of it, and if this book can be a tiny stepping-stone to that, it would be a miracle for us. People with fibromyalgia need to talk about it. The more we talk about it, the more interest and research will be directed our way. God has a reason for giving each of us this illness and our purpose is very important. Just because we don't know what the reasons are now, doesn't mean it was an accident or that we are being punished. He's put this story in my heart and in the hands of others with fibromyalgia right now in hopes that it will touch us in a positive way. We must keep our heads up. This is a battle we can win.

Chapter Three: Vicki, My Mom

My, where have the last seven years gone? At the time we were experiencing them, they just crept by. I'm so glad we have finally evolved into the "good" years. As a mother, it's hard to recap all that Kara has gone through. It's like a bad nightmare that I don't want to relive, but if it can help others survive through their trials, then it's worth the resurfacing of history.

In the beginning, individual symptoms showed up, and we treated them as isolated injuries. But after the first year, it seemed the injuries just kept multiplying and the traditional medical treatments didn't seem to take care of them. As parents, we continued to seek out anyone who might help her. Our family doctor reached his limitation, and referring to a specialist was the next step. Each additional rung on the ladder offered additional hope to us. We were eager to try another approach, although it often meant more medications. The specialist's suggestions resulted in very little improvement. It was frustrating when Kara would wake up with extreme pain, (Pick a spot; it could surface anywhere!) and we'd take her to the E.R. to only find out three to four hours later that they couldn't find anything wrong. Or we'd greet her in the morning to discover that she hadn't been able to sleep all night. I recall her rheumatologist even admitting her to the hospital overnight to assist in sleeping and controlling the pain. I spent the night with her, and, even with the stronger medications, she didn't sleep well. I felt helpless. A mother is supposed to take care of her children's needs, and I couldn't even help my daughter sleep through the night or live a day without pain.

Through these last seven years, Kara and I have visited dozens of doctors and have heard many theories on treating fibromyalgia. We learned a little bit from each doctor, but also discovered that they are just as frustrated with this illness as we are. We also found that every sufferer is individual. What works for one person may not work for someone else. We became very open to holistic methods when we found the traditional methods weren't exactly working. Kara is so much stronger mentally now that she has been able to eliminate many of her medications. This has, in turn, decreased the side effects she suffered in addition to the daily chronic pain.

I feel so much more at ease at this stage of Kara's life. She has gained so much strength from her journey. She's fine-tuning the treatment for her illness and is now able to enjoy life with fewer "bad" days. We still talk often on the phone. Her dad and I always joke each day about whether we've received the "Karrot call" yet. Usually, we both have! Thank goodness for cell phones. We learned through these years to never give up and always be available, day or night, to help our child. With our faith and close family bond, we chose to never let this take control of our lives.

Chapter Four

Fibromyalgia is one of the most frustrating disorders doctors are facing these days. It is not only frustrating to the doctors but also unimaginably frustrating to the people who suffer from it. There isn't a great amount known about fibromyalgia. There isn't one blood test that tells if you have it, not one tell-tale sign, not one specific symptom that can immediately diagnose this illness. It's almost impossible to tell if someone has fibromyalgia just by looking at them, and it's even more impossible to know their pain and suffering because there is no standard way to gauge it. The road to diagnosis is a long and grueling one and can sometimes take years. It's mostly a process of elimination to see what illnesses you don't have. If all the tests come back without incident, it's called fibromyalgia, the catchall. No one wants to be diagnosed with fibromyalgia because the treatments for it are so weak and there has been almost an unmentionable amount of research done for the syndrome. Some people think because they have an ache or a pain that they have fibromyalgia. That's frustrating to people who really do have fibromyalgia because doctors see so many people who claim they have it that when they finally see someone who does, they are so fed up with hearing about it that they don't give us the time of day.

I'm not speaking as an expert about fibromyalgia. I'm speaking as one who experiences it everyday. It has to be quite frustrating for the medical field to research an illness they have no way of understanding. I think it's up to those with fibromyalgia to talk about it and for the world to pay attention to this serious illness. This matter needs to be taken into our own hands. If we don't act, I'm not sure who will.

As I've said, I'm not trying to come across as an expert on fibromyalgia by any means, although sometimes I feel like I know more than the doctors I visit. I feel like I've taken every single traditional medical approach there is: physical therapy, drugs, rheumatologists, pain specialists, and psychologists. I have been left with little but frustration and anger. Not that they haven't helped any, but I knew they weren't my answer.

I've taught yoga for four years and have become very aware and interested in holistic therapies. The most success I've found is through chiropractic and massage. But most importantly, I found a holistic medical doctor who has really emphasized the importance of nutrition, mineral supplements, food allergies, and spiritual balance. I can't possibly say enough about how much she's changed my life. She took the time to go through my entire medical history and just dig in to find any clues about why I was having these issues. She ordered tests that no other doctor had ever even mentioned and showed a level of caring and genuine concern that I'd never experienced with any other doctor. She discovered I had food allergies and mineral deficiencies that might have been causing a lot of my symptoms. As a result, with her heaven sent guidance, I've made changes to my diet and medicine intake that have made my quality of life increase drastically. The moral of the story is, just don't give up. You will find someone who can help you. Be open-minded, and don't ever give up.

Chapter Five

Being diagnosed with any illness, I think, is like a death–the death of a person you thought you were, who you thought you could be, the part of you that didn't have to take medications and see doctors constantly. That person is gone, done. Friendships change for the better or worse. The ones meant to be in your life stay and the ones you thought were meant to be in your life fade out. I thank God I have the parents and siblings that I do because they always believed me. They read, researched, and talked to anyone that could help me and never gave up on getting "their Kara" back. I know, without their love and support, I wouldn't have had the strength or the courage to fight this.

I am fortunate enough to have a family that let me grieve, and they were open about grieving with and for me. In my experience, this is such an important time to go through. I had to have anger and confusion and sadness and questions about God. I had to get it out or it would have killed me. I'm sort of a proud person, and asking for help isn't always easy for me. But I could not do this alone. I tried and tried, but a person can only handle so much. I had to learn to take advantage of the people who want to help me. It made me feel better and saved my loved ones from feeling like they were just watching me suffer.

As I've mentioned before, I've had tattered relationships because of this illness, not only because it was difficult for others to understand, but because it's a big part of my life and who I am. If I can't talk about it with someone when I need to, I'm not giving that person Kara. They are only getting a piece, and that isn't fair to either of us. For good or bad, fibromyalgia has molded me into the person I am today.

A few years ago, I met a man named Randi. He was a friend of a friend, and for a couple years we occasionally chatted and kept in touch. He's beautiful on the outside, but more so on the inside. Caring, confident, motivated, he's someone I just couldn't help but want to be around. I don't remember the exact moment when I knew I loved him. It came on kind of slowly, like all good things seem to.

As fate would have it, a few years after we met, we ended up moving to neighboring towns. We drew closer, and I knew that he really was someone special, someone I could confide in. I told him right away about my illness, I didn't want to waste his time or mine if it wasn't something he could deal with. He said," Ok, what can I do to help," and has been saying it ever since.

I still remember our first kiss, when he told me he loved me, and our first date. One of his best traits is that he just loves me. Plain and simple, not wanting anything back, he realizes my limits. He knows when to push me and when to let me rest.

I've never been able to be as open as I am with him in any other relationships. He just gets it. It didn't come easily; we had to work on it, but he actually made an effort because being with me was that important to him. He asks perfect questions. "What do you want me to do when you're sick?" "What do you want me to say?" "What are good things to say and bad things to say?"

He's also been very honest with me about how hard it is for him. I appreciate that because it's something we go through together. Instead of keeping things bottled up, we've both learned that in order for us to work, we have to talk openly and honestly.

He's told me when he thinks my medication is changing my personality, which I welcome because I'm kind of removed from that aspect. I'm just waiting for something to perk me up, and he knows who I really am and what I really act like enough to know that maybe a medication isn't the one I should be on. He feels comfortable enough with me to say, "I know you feel awful right now, but I need you to listen to me." I'm so grateful to him for being so real with me because I would never know. We can talk it out, and it ends up bringing us closer. Sometimes I just get so trapped in my own bubble.

He keeps me accountable. When I'm cranky he urges me to sleep. He will remind me we need to not stay out late so I can get to bed. He always chooses to lay low and watch movies when he might rather go out. It's hard work, but it's so worth it. To mentally survive, I have to have a few people I can totally empty myself to. I think it makes them feel better, so they aren't always wondering, *What should I be doing to help?*

Chapter Six: Randi

I've known Kara for almost five years. We recently got engaged and will marry in the summer of 2007. I'll never forget the first date I had with Kara. She invited me over to her place for dinner. I was having a great time, even though I think Kara would agree when I say I found out right off the bat that fettuccini alfredo isn't her specialty. Later in the evening, when we were watching a movie, I noticed Kara seemed uncomfortable. It appeared that she was either in a lot of pain, or not having a good time. I didn't know what to think. I *thought* that we were having a great time. Clearly I couldn't have been *that* bad of a date. I had cleaned up nicely, put on the least wrinkled shirt I could find, tried my hardest to make her laugh, and even pretended to enjoy every bite of the food she had so diligently prepared for us. So it came as a shock to me that this girl sitting beside me seemed so miserable. I never considered myself to have a way with women, but I couldn't figure this one out.

I asked her if something was wrong and she started explaining to me, in a nutshell, her story. She told me that she was having a "flare-up" and that she was hurting pretty badly. In short, a completely foreign word was added to my vocabulary that night: fibromyalgia. I had never heard of it before, and I knew nothing about it. I listened to more of what Kara said, and I couldn't believe what she was telling me. Could a young, beautiful girl that appeared to be completely healthy have such a debilitating chronic disorder? Surely this couldn't be the case.

Chronic illnesses and pain syndromes are what elderly people get, not a girl like Kara in the prime of her young adult life! So the night ended, and although Kara may have thought she'd never see me again, she did. She's been stuck with me ever since.

When Kara asked me to write something for this story, I was hesitant. I haven't been here from the beginning and didn't know nearly as much about the situation as her parents do. I thought about it awhile and finally decided that if Kara was brave enough to write such a graphic, personal book about herself, the least I could do was contribute what I could. I can attest to what I see as significant progress in her overall condition. I don't think this progress is because her illness is going away, but rather, due to how she deals with her condition and takes care of herself on a daily basis.

I think one of the hardest things I've ever dealt with has been seeing someone I love so much in constant pain and thinking there's nothing I can do to help. True, I can't "fix" the pain, but I've found out there is something I can do that helps – listen. I think, many times, all someone with fibromyalgia wants is to talk to someone, to let them know how they're feeling and not have to keep it in all the time.

In order to listen, I have to believe when Kara tells me she's hurting. No matter what any doctor of psychiatrist says or what any test shows (or doesn't show), I always believe Kara. The biggest mistake I can make is to doubt her. I owe it to the person I love to support every possible approach, technique, philosophy, and crazy off-the-wall remedy there is out there until we find something that helps. Even if that means going against "mainstream health-care." Kara has run into more than her share of closed-minded, ignorant, arrogant doctors, many of whom don't seem to have a clue what fibromyalgia is or even care to know. Fibromyalgia sufferers and their families need to live by one motto: if someone can't help you or doesn't believe you, then find someone who will.

I think a number of things have helped Kara fight to improve, or at least come to terms with her condition. First of all, she's one of the toughest and most resilient people I know. She never quits. She keeps going every day and does what she has to do to make it though that day. Second, Kara's accepted that she can't do things other people can do or that she used to do. However, I think she's found out that there are many things she's capable of doing that she never realized before getting sick. Kara's faith and spirituality have also kept her going through some of the harder times. Finally, Kara has amazing support from her entire family. She couldn't ask for a more loving family who would drop everything and do anything for her at a moment's notice.

I've tried my hardest to help Kara any way I can, but I'll admit it's very difficult sometimes. I've learned through mistakes and trial and error, I guess. Sometimes I just have to accept that there's nothing I can do except listen and be there for her. It's one of the hardest things I've ever had to do. I know I have to stay positive as much as possible. Kara has had to be realistic and accept the fact that she may never be totally "cured." I know Kara gets frustrated when people promise her relief or the magic remedy and can't back it up. But what I love about Kara is she never gives up. She takes it one day at a time and knows her limits. She keeps trying new therapies, new doctors, new exercise plans, and new diets, anything and everything to help her feel better. And I think she is seeing some dividends from her patience and determination.

Chapter Seven

The first productive place I went, after my family doctor admitted he didn't know what else to do for me, was an amazing rheumatologist. He seemed untouched by the day-in and day-out repetition of his job. He was very calming and gentle. He wasn't questioning the validity of my pain the way previous doctors had. He was asking me questions instead of my parents. He made sure I felt in control and that I had a say in what was happening. I didn't care what he was going to tell me. I knew something was wrong, and I was so tired of doctors telling me just because my blood tests came back normal, nothing was wrong with me. I didn't care what they called the illness. I just desperately needed help.

He told us there were a few things they were testing for. I almost prayed that I would be diagnosed with one of them so someone would finally believe me and know what to do to help me. He mentioned lupus, rheumatoid arthritis, leukemia, juvenile arthritis, fibromyalgia and a few others. I didn't know much about any of them except they were all very serious.

The tests showed everything was fine, so they threw me into the catchall illness: fibromyalgia. I knew nothing about it. I started to research it, but the personal stories and websites I found weren't much help. It didn't seem like there was going to be any relief in the future. We had a name, but really, nothing else. I began an aggressive regimen of pain and sleeping medicine. The next couple months were a blur. I wasn't functioning like myself anymore. I was constantly sleepy and groggy feeling. I didn't have any emotions towards anything. I was numb to the world. It was like I was walking around and going through the motions physically, but mentally, I wasn't even in the room. Along with the pain, I had been diagnosed with depression, anxiety, and obsessive compulsive disorder, all of which I believe were indicative to my situation.

It became extremely hard to hide my diagnosis from friends and teachers. It was obvious that something was wrong with me, but no one knew what it was. I didn't want anyone to know because I thought they wouldn't believe me. I was a tough athlete, a girl other kids looked up to. I could make it through this. *I'm not going to let some disease that doesn't even show up in the spell check on my computer get me down.* So I pushed it away, refusing to let it wear me down, but as time passed, my physical strength diminished along with my spirit.

Cross-country and track had been a big part of my high school career. It was something I was good at, loved, and worked hard at. I loved to run more than anything. I would come home from practices not feeling like I had worked hard enough and would run a couple extra miles for fun. Running made me feel free, like I could do anything. It was how I dealt with regular teenage life and frustrations.

My junior year was an enormous struggle, mostly because my illness was just becoming apparent and serious, but partially because of my cross-country coach. She caused me a tremendous amount of pain that was really hard to get over. I can usually figure people out right away. I couldn't with her, though. I was just as taken as everyone else by her charisma. The whole team thrived on her praise. I don't know if it was more me than the other girls, but I really loved her. During a race, I could pick her voice out from a huge crowd and use it to push myself. We had a very close team. We were like a family.

I looked up to her so much. I knew that she was my teacher and coach, but I somehow felt that I was more special to her than that. I don't know if I really was. So many kids looked up to her, I think I felt special that she seemed to care about me and our team more than any other students. I believed I was her friend. As far as I was concerned, her word was as good as gold. I always wanted to impress her and make her proud of me. The whole situation seems so messed up when I look back on it now, but at the time that's just the way it was.

Before my fibromyalgia diagnosis, I went to doctors primarily for knee and shoulder pain. They had told me the only way to be rid of my pain was to quit running, that my body just wasn't able to handle it. I'd been very diligent with cortisone shots and physical therapy, but nothing made a bit of difference. I kept this from her for a while, but it was too much for me to handle on my own. When I told her, she knew I would never quit. So she used it as motivation for me. "Prove the doctors wrong. Show them that you are tough and that you can do this." The pain I was going through to run seemed worth it when I got praise from her.

My body was making it impossible for me to put in as many miles as the team did in practice. Coach and I decided that I would ride a bike throughout practice and only run in the meets. I'd leave practice almost unable to walk to my car because of the pain I was in, but determined no one would see my weakness. I iced every night and before and after every race. It was hard, emotionally, on me too. I wanted so badly to run! This was what I loved, and I was a mess knowing sooner or later, I would have to quit for good. The thought of it was too hard to handle, so I just kept pushing it back and pretending I was okay. I was just a puppet, a fake, going through the motions, lying to *everyone, all* the time. Since I didn't get a workout going the same pace as my team, I would end up riding my bike ahead by myself. It was lonely, but I was determined not to let myself or anyone else down. When they were out running the five-mile block and saw me breezing past on my bike, I knew they thought I was faking it and grumbled at my stupid bike and me.

I was working so hard. I woke up one morning and couldn't even lift myself up to look at my clock. I was so fatigued and in so much pain that I literally couldn't even get out of bed. I missed a meet that day. I was taking way to much pain medicine just to get through the day and had developed an ulcer-like pain in my stomach. It was a no-win situation: take the medicine and run, or don't take it and be in pain constantly. My mom called my coach and told her I was sick and wouldn't be at the meet today. I knew she would be upset, but I didn't really have any other choice. My parents had stood by reluctantly while I beat myself up physically and mentally, and I think my mom knew I needed her to put her foot down and tell me she wouldn't let me run that day because I wouldn't have on my own.

The next day was terrible. No one on my team would talk to me except one of my best girlfriends. I couldn't even imagine the kinds of things Coach had said about me. I was too scared to even talk to her. I was terrified of what she was going to say to me, and I felt I deserved everything she was going to say to me.

I passed her once in the hallway, and she blatantly ignored me. So after school I went and asked her if there was something we needed to talk about. I honestly have never felt so helpless and humiliated in my entire life. We lost the first place title because I wasn't there to place. One of the other girls was running with shin splints, and I couldn't even get through a stomachache. I'd let everyone down. It was all my fault.

She was so mad at me; she said she didn't even want to look at me. I just stood there and took it all. I believed her. Everything she said, I believed. I knew it was my fault and was mad at myself for not having sucked it up and ran. I tried feebly at first to defend myself, but I knew it was a lost cause. I was red-faced and crying. She told me to get dressed and meet her out on the course. I said, "No, I quit."

She kind of laughed and challenged, "You'd never quit." I wanted so badly to run home, to cry to my mom and tell her the awful thing that had just happened to me, to hide safely in my bed. I didn't, though; I stood there with my hands turning white from my tight fists and my jaw aching from my clenched teeth and didn't move. She told me to hurry up and change and meet her out on the practice course. The team was waiting for me to apologize. I cried the entire practice. She was right. I was too weak.

The next year, after having an extremely difficult summer that forced me to quit softball. I didn't go out for cross-country. My body just couldn't handle it. Coach told just about everyone that would listen, it seemed, that I was quitting because I wanted to drink or party. I don't really know all the things that she said about me. Honestly, I don't really care. I didn't have the energy or care enough to correct her. I was seventeen and diagnosed with fibromyalgia and didn't know what to say to anyone. I just let her and everyone else come to their own conclusions about why I wasn't running anymore: hurt knees, differences with the coach, boyfriend, whatever. I didn't correct anyone. I didn't have the energy and didn't think anyone would believe me anyway.

Finally, years later, I've come to a place where I can forgive her. We've talked, not necessarily about what happened, but we've talked. I know she feels a lot of guilt over what happened once she found out what was going on with me. It wasn't her fault, but I felt like she was the first person who left me when I started getting sick. She didn't know what was wrong with me, and there were people to come who wouldn't understand what I was going through and would give up. It just reaffirmed to me that I couldn't tell anyone what was happening to me because they wouldn't believe me. I guess it's not as hard to deal with the second and third time someone leaves you, but the first is always the hardest to get over.

Chapter Eight: Bryan, My Dad

I always hoped to be that dad who could fix almost anything. Taking care of my wife and kids is my real job, and I take it very seriously. Gosh, I can fix a broken bike, shingle a roof, teach a good jump shot, plumb the sink, and make a skinned knee feel better. My kids know that they can come to me for anything, and I will take care of it. That is, until we discovered Kara had fibromyalgia.

The "discovery" has been a journey of pain, speculation, doctors of various specialties, kooks with everything from a prayer to a vitamin, frustration, depression, and an experiment in pharmacology.

Kara, as a youngster and early teen, was as normal as all kids: active, cheery, social, and, by all means, a normal well-adjusted girl. From as early as seventh grade, Kara was very interested in running. She just loved to run. Her other passion was to be a catcher for the high school softball team. She liked sports, and she was good at them. It was not uncommon for her to come home from track or cross-country practice and go running again. Kara was a varsity track star as a freshman and a state cross-country runner as well.

In her sophomore year, there were what we thought natural athletic injuries: aches and pains, sore knees, and sore shoulders at first. Anti-inflammatory, Tylenol, cold and warm packs, and even cortisone shots were the therapeutic modalities. The relief was very temporary and probably psychosomatic. We just prayed something would make things feel better.

I wanted so to find the solution, but this pain was not normal and very much out of our control. *Why can't we fix this? Is it real? How many doctors do we have to talk to before we have something to hold on to? Why can't I fix this? I'm supposed to be able to take care of her!* So, the spiral began! Over the course of a year, I was seeing my very active, athletic daughter go down hill before my very eyes. The very things that she loved and was good at became impossible for her.

No more cross country; no more track; no more softball. This athletic, muscle-toned kid was no more. *What's going on? Why can't we get some answers?* I could tell that she was becoming very depressed, and I couldn't fix that either.

I remember sitting in the rheumatologist's office with a photo in my hand and tears in my eyes, pleading with the doctor for help. "Look at his picture," I told the doctor. "Look at the legs of this athlete and then look at my daughter now! Please help her. I think I'm losing my daughter right before my eyes! I don't know what else to do."

I loved watching Kara run. She was beautiful. I loved the effort and the drive. I always thought you could really find out what a kid was made of by watching her run a long race. No matter what the place, the effort to compete and finish that race was something to behold. That determination and drive would come in handy during this long and confusing journey.

In this journey of ours, we turned our hope to a dizzying number and specialty of doctors. I can't tell you how many times we researched and chose *another* doctor. We'd wait on the appointment date with great anticipation and hope that this may be the one. When the wait was over, there was almost always this unbelievable let down. Again, no help, again, more drugs, again, some asshole who *disregards* this kid who's dealing with unceasing, merciless pain. I can't imagine the disappointment and desperation that my Kara has endured.

I believe that doctors can be divided into categories on this issue. There are doctors who try to help but just don't know what to do. There are doctors who *say* they know exactly what to do and absolutely don't. And there are doctors who don't believe that this pain or condition exists and disregard this desperate patient as a psychiatric patient.

I am a person of faith. God will not give a person more than what they can handle. I truly believe this, but I also believe for some reason, God may push a person to the very brink. Yes, I believe that Kara was standing on a razor's edge between life and death. The very thought of this kind of desperation in my loved one grips my heart with a pain that cannot be adequately described. It's the very God and faith that tests us to the brink that also has the power and love to bring us to the light. Kara has endured this test. She is a better person for her trials. Her courage has been tested. Her faith has be tested and ultimately strengthened by this journey. She is so beautiful inside and out. With some hesitation, I can say that I believe this condition in many ways has made her the great person she is today.

I have described some of the darkness and desperation that has come with this condition. When we found that rare doctor who would listen, understand, and treat Kara, we knew we had a real jewel. The darkness became light. Now there is real and understandable hope for Kara. Her pain still exists but is greatly eased. She is no longer on a long list of painkillers and antidepressants. Kara has fought and worked very hard on her current life of strength, less pain, and stronger faith. Life is much better, thanks to a doctor who cared enough to help.

The final component that is key to Kara's survival is a family that learned to believe and understand. Kara has a mother who could not give up and has been available at any minute of the day to talk or go to her, no matter the miles or time. She has siblings who showed understanding and tolerance for the energy that all this takes. We are family, and nothing, no one, will stand between us.

Chapter Nine

Near the end of my senior year of high school, when graduation was the only thing on everyone's mind, I found myself in a tailspin. Everything was getting out of control. I didn't eat or sleep. My appetite was non-existent, and becoming thinner and thinner somehow made me feel good, or in control. When I was in very good shape, weight lifting, and healthy, I was five-foot-four, one-hundred-twenty pounds, and thin. I didn't have extra weight to lose.

A few weeks after graduation, I was below ninety-eight pounds. I looked sick, terribly sick and weak. My clothes didn't fit anymore. Everything hung off me and looked two sizes too big. My mom and dad had resorted to having me write down, every day, everything I ate, every medicine I took, my hours of sleep, and what my body felt like that day. Of course I lied about that too, not wanting to make a fuss, not wanting anyone to ask questions.

I wasn't anorexic; I didn't care enough about myself to eat. Maybe that is anorexia. I don't know. I didn't care what other people thought about me. My family and friends seemed sickened by my appearance. Everyone made comments about it. I felt like my family was more embarrassed than anything when people asked, but I know that they were just worried and didn't know what to do. They would talk about it all the time, always asking if I had eaten anything today. I liked that people asked about my weight and not about why I was sick or had quit sports. I always lied. I lied about everything. That's what I did. I lied to everyone about how I was feeling, why I was crying. The truth took too much energy and was too hard to talk about. I didn't feel like anyone would believe or understand me. I felt like a fake. I was this whole different person who no one even knew about. If I didn't eat anything all day, I was excited. It was something I could do without anyone knowing, and I didn't have to listen to anyone else. I was being tough in a different way. Mentally, I thought I was being strong and disciplined by starving myself, which made me feel I was making up for my lack of physical strength. Getting thin was just my positive reinforcement, like winning a race. I felt I had to regain control over something and I thought I was being "successful."

Chapter Ten

That was the beginning of the end of the most intense period of my coming to terms with fibromyalgia. The rest of that summer and a few years into my college life, I used alternative ways to cope with my frustration and pain–not many of which I'm proud of. I drank to numb-out physically and mentally, was extremely suicidal at times, carelessly and dangerously used prescription pain medication, self-mutilated, didn't eat, and lost myself in pointless and destructive relationships.

I can remember distinctly a time when I was eighteen and I was so depressed hours would just fly by and I wouldn't even notice. I literally would just sit in my room and stare at the wall. I could hear my sister's playing basketball outside, I heard the neighbors mowing their lawns, heard the phone ring, but I just stayed sitting there. Finally I got up went into the kitchen, dumped two bottles of pills in my hand. I rolled them around with the fingers of my other hand, thought about how much water it would take to swallow all the pills. My hands were shaking and I was crying. When the pills were close enough to my mouth to smell I got so freaked out I poured them all back in the bottle, slammed the cabinet door, grabbed the phone and ran to my room. I called my dad in hysterics telling him that if he didn't come home I was scared what I would do to myself.

When I look back at those times in my life, it makes me feel very lonely. I mourn for that girl who was so lost and scared. I still didn't really have people other than my family to talk to about my feelings. There was still a lot of grief and anger that was just festering and boiling beneath my surface.

People have asked me how could I ever think about or do such terrible things to myself, but I honestly felt that I had to punish myself for not being who I thought I was supposed to be. I felt real relief when I put myself in pain by cutting because at least I could control that pain. I couldn't control the fibromyalgia pain. I couldn't even get medical doctors to believe me. I hadn't figured out who I was with this illness yet. I was still battling it, trying to win a war that couldn't ever be won. As I've gotten older, I've learned better. Not many people knew that I had those problems, so it was something I just worked out on my own, with credit due to my therapist also. I was too embarrassed to let anyone know that I'd gotten that pathetic. It's all about trial and error. Sometimes I'm so thick-headed and try so hard to fit in with people my age by going out to bars, but even the very few times I do it, I know how crappy I'm going to feel. This illness has forced me to grow up a lot quicker that I would have. Usually I make the right choices, but once in a while I try to be my age, knowing full well that that's not my life.

Chapter Eleven

As recently as last year, before I found my now-coveted holistic doctor, I was still experiencing a lot of daily pain. Not sleeping, I knew my quality of life could be better, had to be better because I wasn't satisfied with living that way. I had a previous doctor mention that maybe I should try to get into the University pain clinic. I thought it was a great idea, an approach I hadn't yet tried. I needed a referral from a rheumatologist, and I didn't think that was going to be a problem at all, just a stepping-stone. As it turned out, there was a two-month-long waiting list to get into this particular rheumatologist, so while I waited, I researched the pain clinic and felt some tentative hope. It seemed like the pain clinic could be helpful to me. They had treated people with fibromyalgia.

I was excited to see this doctor because I was certain he would give me the referral that I needed and had once again let myself get hopeful that I could find some relief. I was careful, though, because I'd experienced many letdowns. It just seemed like a cycle of ups and downs, and I thought I had gotten past the point where I actually expected something good to happen at the doctor's office, but I just had to have something to look forward to. My reality was driving me crazy.

This doctor had come pretty highly recommended, and I thought his waiting list was an indication of how good he was. It wasn't. I had been very insistent that every record in reference to my diagnosis from any hospital I'd ever been to had been at his disposal, so he had read from at least four different doctors, confirming my fibromyalgia diagnosis.

He came in, took a look at my chart, checked the eighteen tender points, and, after a five-minute assessment, made up his mind. He said I didn't have stable joints, that they were too loose. He asked me to touch my ear to my shoulder, and when I couldn't do that, he told me I must not be that good of a yoga instructor. After looking at the antidepressants and various medications I was on, he said that the reason I hurt was because I was too depressed and couldn't sleep. He said I didn't have fibromyalgia and that, "your other doctors were wrong and just didn't know what else to tell you anymore." His solution was to go back to my psychiatrist and get "a much stronger" antidepressant. He said I would feel better very soon. My pain would go away, and that was that.

I was dumbfounded, just absolutely stunned. I said, "So every other doctor that I've gone to has been misdiagnosing me along the way?" His answer was, "Yes, you need Prozac" and that I had believed it because I was depressed. Near tears, I'm sure I affirmed to him that I was depressed. He was probably thinking, "I'm so smart for helping her." I just couldn't think of anything to say. He wasn't going to refer me to the pain clinic because he felt he'd fixed that problem by sending me back to my psychiatrist. I couldn't even get him to refill a pain medication I'd been taking for years. I'd been insulted and treated like I was crazy, but he told me he had a video that I should watch before I left. He thought it would be helpful to me, maybe give me some tips.

I just kind of went along with it, thinking it was going to be something on teenage depression. The video was from 1983, titled, "Fibromyalgia. What is it? How to deal with your diagnosis and what to do next."

I was completely crushed. I was so mad I walked out without paying. *He doesn't deserve to get paid.* Of course I knew they would bill me, but it made me feel better to just leave. I got to my car, and the tears were already turned on to the max. It was just so simple for him. *I've been dealing with this for years and years, and you see me for ten minutes and just turn everything upside down.* I thought I had gotten past the point where doctors could make me feel like that. I thought I was tougher than that. I didn't think it was possible for a doctor, a rheumatologist especially, to tell me this was all in my head again. *In 2005, with fibromyalgia making its way more and more into offices and you just dismiss everything every previous doctor has told me and documented, then, after telling me I don't have fibromyalgia, have the nerve to sit me down and watch a movie about an illness I supposedly don't have?* I was mad and just disappointed. What was I going to do now? I couldn't believe after everything I'd been through, that I was back to square one with this man telling me it was all in my head.

It just made me sick that he was going to walk out of his office and probably forget about me the second he saw his next patient and have no idea the damage he had just done to me. I called my mom and fiancé, almost unable to talk because I was crying so much, wondering out loud if it really was in my head. "Am I doing this to myself?" Of course, I knew better, and they reassured me that he was a terrible doctor and that we would just find someone else. But right then I promised myself I would never go to a conventional doctor again regarding my fibromyalgia. I haven't since then and don't plan on it.

Chapter Twelve

I've been writing about all this for five years. The moments that I've shared have been some of the lowest I've ever experienced. I share them because I know the comfort I receive when I know that I don't have to feel alone. I've learned such an enormous amount about myself, about the resiliency of the human spirit, and about healing. When I started writing this, I was very angry, young, and just trying to find out how I was going to fit into a world where most young adults don't have a chronic illness. Now, I finally feel like I'm a woman and that I'm to a point where I can handle what God has given me with strength and grace.

Over the years, my spectrum of fibromyalgia acquaintances has grown and taught me more than I could imagine. Now, I'm a certified yoga instructor and currently working on my degree in Therapeutic Recreation to help those who are also chronically ill. I came to this path and occupation through my need for personal healing and a sense that I could somehow, hopefully, make a small difference. Through yoga, I've worked with a lot of women who are chronically ill or also dealing with fibromyalgia. It's the most rewarding thing I've ever done in my life. There are a lot of women worse off than me, and when they call me an inspiration to them, I don't think I've ever gotten a compliment that means so much.

Sometimes I think about the time at that dead-end road, when I was feeling so low and alone. People talk about hitting rock bottom. That really was it for me; it scares me to think of how many times I truly thought suicide was my only escape. I've always believed in God. I've always believed that there is a higher power that we all answer to. At the time, I couldn't figure out why I was left all alone, why I couldn't pick myself up off the floor. How could God see me in that much pain and do nothing? But he wasn't doing nothing. I realize, now, that that moment, one that I thought was the worst in my life, wasn't. God was there. He was everywhere. If I had never had the chance to feel that sort of raw agony, desperation, and fear, I couldn't be able to see the beauty of my life now.

Thank You

The emotional strength it has taken to write this book has only been possible through the support of my friends and family.

My parents, Bryan and Vicki, you've never wavered in your support and belief in me. You are both my rock, my safe place. Thank you to my siblings Justyn, Kristyn, and Jenny for your acceptance, understanding, and for being my best friends. Thank you Randi, you are my heart and perfect better half. Also thanks to Laura, Amanda, Libby, Sarah, Rachel, Gia, Dr. Karyn Shanks, and many others who truly listen. Lastly, I thank God for giving me the courage to have a voice.

About the Author

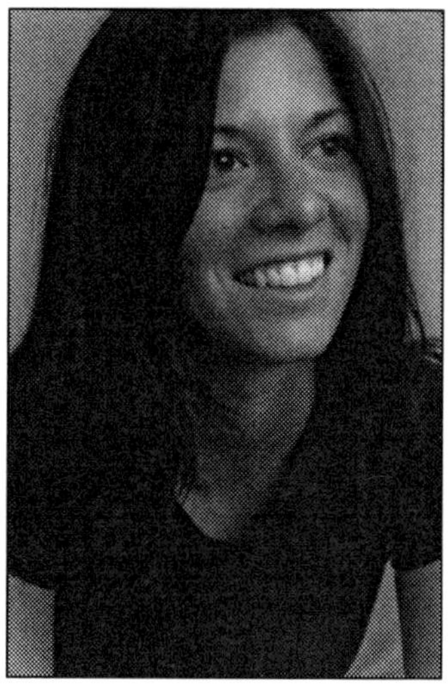

Kara lives in Iowa and enjoys yoga, reading, and spending time with family and friends.

Lightning Source UK Ltd.
Milton Keynes UK
29 December 2009

147975UK00001B/104/A

9 781595 266170